HADLEY VLAHOS BOOK

A HOSPICE NURSE WITH A HEART OF GOLD

TIM PATRICK MOSS

Table of Content

INTRODUCTION

Hadley Vlahos has witnessed a number of deaths that surpasses people's imagination. Being a hospice nurse, she has dedicated hours at the bedside of patients nearing the end providing them with solace, care and understanding. However, amidst her experiences Hadley has also learned lessons that have inspired her to embrace life more authentically and appreciatively.

Within this biography lies the extraordinary tale of Hadley Vlahos—a journey that begins with her origins as a sensitive child and culminates in her pursuit of becoming a nurse, author and influential figure on social media. Furthermore, this biography offers glimpses into the realm of hospice care; its challenges, its power on those who partake in it.

Not solely focused on honoring Hadley Vlahos and her exceptional contributions, this biography delves into contemplations surrounding life's meaning and purpose in relation to death. It delves into themes such as love, loss, grief, hope, faith and joy—the very threads interwoven into the tapestry of Hadley's existence and vocation. Moreover, this narrative shares the messages and wisdom bestowed upon Hadley by her patients—messages of inspiring and enlightening all who encounter them.

Ultimately this biography serves as an ode to Hadley Vlahos—her moments bridging the gap between life and death—a tribute that reveals both beauty and mystery inherent, within these moments.

It's a tale that will deeply move you, stimulate your thoughts and ignite your spirit.

Chapter 1

Early Life and Education

Vlahos came into this world on June 12, 1993 in Baton Rouge, Louisiana. She was the youngest of three siblings and the only daughter of John and Mary Vlahos. Her parents owned a restaurant that brought them much success. Growing up Hadley experienced the warmth and support of her knit family, which included her parents, brothers, grandparents, aunts, uncles and cousins.

During her years Hadley's life was shaped by her grandparent's profession, as embalmers and funeral directors. They operated a family-owned funeral home where Hadley often accompanied them and offered assistance.

Witnessing the rituals and ceremonies surrounding death captivated her interest. She developed a reverence for honoring the deceased and their families while also gaining experience, with grief and compassion.

As a child Hadley possessed introversion coupled with sensitivity; she found solace in books writing rather than participating in sports or social gatherings. Her imaginative mind overflowed with creativity as she nurtured aspirations of becoming an author one day.

Hadley went to a school until she turned ten years old where she received a strict religious education. They taught her about God, heaven, hell, angels and demons. Emphasized following the church's rules and doctrines. She was an obedient student who regularly prayed and attended church services every week.

However, when Hadley reached fifteen years old, a tragic event shook her faith to its core. Her closest friend Sarah passed away in a car accident leaving Hadley devastated and full of questions. She couldn't comprehend why God would take away someone young and innocent while seemingly ignoring her pleas for intervention. These circumstances led her to question everything she had been taught and doubt the existence of God's benevolence.

This crisis of faith caused tension between Hadley and her family – with her religious parents. They tried their best to console her while simultaneously pressuring her to return to the church fold and accept it as God's plan. They disapproved of her exploration of beliefs or perspectives fearing that she might be losing herself.

Feeling isolated and misunderstood, Hadley sought solace in writing as an alternative for her emotions. She began writing in a journal pouring out her thoughts and emotions while expressing her uncertainties and anxieties. She also delved into the realms of poetry and storytelling exploring themes such, as life, death, love, loss and faith. Writing became her solace and therapy helping her navigate through grief and confusion.

In addition to writing Hadley found companionship and support among a group of individuals who shared her sense of curiosity and skepticism. They introduced her to perspectives encompassing philosophy, literature, music, art as well as substances and they also inspired her to pursue her passion.

Hadley's rebellious phase lingered until she completed school when she encountered another turning point in life. Subsequently moving out from her parents' home, Hadley enrolled herself in nursing school with hopes of finding stability alongside a fulfilling career. With honors Hadley successfully completed nursing school. Began working as a registered nurse in settings including immediate care facilities, nursing homes and hospitals. Through gaining experience in her profession, she earned respect, from both colleagues and patients. During this time she continued to pursue writing by submitting poems and stories to publications and contests.

However it wasn't until she started working in hospice care that Hadley discovered her calling and purpose. She was assigned to provide care in the homes of patients who were in their advanced stages of their life and to offer support to their families during this time. Initially she felt hesitant and anxious about this responsibility. Soon realized that it brought her the fulfillment and purpose she had ever experienced.

Hadley formed lasting connections with her patients, who entrusted her with their stories, regrets, hopes and wisdom. Through them she learned lessons on living embracing gratitude and facing mortality with grace, bravery and serenity. In return she shared her stories, insights and empathy with them. Offering solace, closure and moments of joy.

Inspired by these experiences as a hospice nurse, Hadley decided to chronicle her encounters in a bid to reach an audience. She created an account where she posted videos discussing hospice care alongside the profound lessons imparted by her patients. Additionally

she penned a memoir titled "The In Between; Unforgettable Encounters During Life's Final Moments " delving deeper into her stories, reflections and how they transformed her perspective on life.

As fate would have it Hadley's TikTok account and memoir garnered popularity captivating millions of followers and readers. She received admiration, gratitude, from individuals of all ages and backgrounds who were moved and inspired by her stories and wisdom. However, she also faced criticism and opposition from some individuals who accused her of exploiting and sensationalizing her patients and their families as violating their privacy and dignity.

In response to the controversy Hadley clarified that she always obtained consent and permission from her patients and their families before sharing their stories. She emphasized that she consistently respected their wishes, preferences and privacy. Furthermore, she expressed that her objective was not to gain profit or fame; rather it was to raise awareness about hospice care while encouraging discussions about death and advance care planning. She sincerely hoped that through her stories and messages people would be able to live lives while facing the end. Moreover, she believed that such conversations would foster connections among individuals.

As a result of her success and popularity Hadley found herself facing opportunities as well as challenges. She was invited to speak at events on platforms like podcasts, radio shows, TV shows, TEDx talks. Additionally a major publisher approached her for a book deal while a Hollywood studio offered her a movie deal.

She agreed to these offers. She also experienced the pressure and stress of meeting deadlines and expectations as well as finding a balance between her professional and personal life.

Hadley also married another hospice nurse named Ryan who shared her passion and vision for care. They expanded their family with two children; a daughter named Lily and a son named Leo. They decided to move to a house outside of New Orleans. While Hadley continued working as a hospice nurse, she also dedicated time and effort towards her writing and public speaking career. Additionally, she initiated an organization called Hadley House. The organization's mission was to establish and operate a hospice house that would provide families and patients with comfort and support during their old days.

Chapter 2

Career and Achievements

For ten years Hadley Vlahos has dedicated herself to being a hospice nurse offering in home care to terminally ill patients and their loved ones. She considers it an honor and a privilege to be present during the intimate moments of life and death. Hadley also utilizes her storytelling talent to educate others about the importance of hospice care aiming to make an impact on the world.

However, Hadley's work is not without its share of challenges. She faces emotional, mental and spiritual demands that put her resilience and compassion to the test. Additionally, she encounters obstacles that hinder her ability to provide care for her patients and their families.

Some of the difficulties Hadley confronts as a hospice nurse include;

The persistent shortage of nursing professionals; Hospice care requires the clock attention from individuals who can meet the unique needs and preferences of patients and families. Unfortunately, there is a shortage of nurses including those specializing in hospice care. Contributing factors include wages, high turnover rates, burnout concerns, limited educational opportunities and societal stigmatization. This implies that Hadley frequently finds herself working hours covering shifts and taking care of more patients than she can handle. These circumstances have an impact on her well-being, health and performance as compromising the quality and safety of the care she provides.

Lack of awareness and appreciation; Individuals, including healthcare professionals, patients, families and policymakers, misunderstands and underutilize hospice care. There are misconceptions and fears surrounding hospice care like it being perceived as giving up or hastening death or only being applicable to cancer patients. Additionally, many people are unaware of the benefits and services that hospice care offers such as pain management, emotional support, spiritual guidance and bereavement care. Consequently, Hadley frequently encounters resistance, denial and hostility from individuals she interacts with. She also has to play the role of an advocate by educating others about hospice care. Furthermore, she faces a lack of recognition and respect from colleagues and superiors who fail to appreciate or comprehend her work.

Legal dilemmas; Hospice care involves litigations, alongside legal judgments that necessitate thoughtful decision making.

Hadley encounters challenges in her role, as a hospice nurse involving matters like informed consent, advance directives decisions about life sustaining treatments, palliative sedation, euthanasia and assisted suicide. These issues often create legal dilemmas for Hadley as she strives to balance her responsibilities with her personal values and the preferences of her patients. Additionally, navigating the policies and regulations governing hospice care – such as eligibility criteria, reimbursement rates and quality standards –

can sometimes influence the choices Hadley can make.

One of the demanding aspects of hospice care is the spiritual toll it takes on Hadley. She must cope with the suffering, loss and death experienced by her patients and their families. At the time she must manage her emotions – including feelings of sadness, anger, guilt, fear and doubt. Supporting grieving families while also dealing with her grief is a part of her role. Furthermore, Hadley must confront questions about mortality and spirituality in order to reaffirm her beliefs and values. To maintain well-being in this challenging environment requires finding coping mechanisms to prevent compassion fatigue or burnout.

Despite these difficulties in their profession, as a hospice nurse Hadley does not. Resent the work she does. She firmly believes that the rewards and joys she experiences in her work far outweigh the difficulties and challenges she encounters. The privilege of caring for patients and their families during their journey fills her with a sense of honor and gratitude. Moreover, she gains insights and wisdom from their stories, which further enriches her life. Sharing these stories with an audience brings her fulfillment as she strives to make a positive impact on the world. For her, hospice care is not a profession; it is also a calling and a mission that demands not expertise but also genuine empathy.

Her social mission; Hadley's fascination with the stories and wisdom from her patients was also driven by her desire to make an impact on the world utilizing her storytelling abilities for the good. She was acutely aware of the environmental challenges our world faces including poverty, inequality, violence, climate change and pandemics. The future of humanity and our planet deeply concerned her igniting a passion within her to actively contribute to solutions and necessary changes. Inspired by emerging movements advocating for rights, social justice and environmental sustainability – she aimed to align herself with these causes. Her intention was to lend support through amplifying their messages using her voice and platform.

Chapter 3

Personal Life and Relationships

Hadley Vlahos has always had an compassionate nature. Growing up in a Louisiana town her family had roots, in the local church. The values instilled in her were to follow the rules and show respect for authority figures. They also encouraged her to consider a career in ministry or education as those paths were seen honorable for a woman of faith.

However, Hadley's interests and questions extended beyond these boundaries. She found joy in reading books and delving into cultures and perspectives. Life's mysteries, the concepts of suffering and joy intrigued her deeply. She longed to explore the world while making an impact on people's lives.

Additionally, certain teachings and practices within her church sparked doubts and disagreements within Hadley—particularly concerning matters of sexuality and gender roles.

During school Hadley met Jake—an individual who shared her thirst for knowledge and exploration. Their friendship quickly blossomed into love. Together they began venturing into aspects of their sexuality despite being fully aware of the associated risks and consequences. While they believed they were careful and responsible, with their choices one day Hadley discovered she was expecting a child.

Fear engulfed Hadley as confusion set in; she felt lost without knowing whom to confide in or what steps to take next. She was fully aware that her parents and the people in her community would be extremely angry and disappointed. She knew that she would face judgment and rejection. She also knew that her dreams and laid plans would crumble in an instant. However, she couldn't deny the fact that she deeply loved Jake and their unborn child and she was determined to keep them both.

Her decision was clear. She needed to confide in Jake. Although he was taken aback and frightened by the news, he stood by her side with unwavering support assuring her of his commitment. Together they made a pact to face their parents as a front ready to bear the consequences. They held onto optimism hoping against hope that their families would comprehend their situation and find it within themselves to forgive them. Their fervent desire was for everyone involved to come and find a resolution.

Reality aligned with their hopes. As they revealed the truth about their situation to their parents, they supported her.

Hadley gathered her belongings and boarded a bus bound for New Orleans hoping for a start. They found an apartment. Began searching for employment. Additionally, they enrolled in a community college to continue her education and pursue their interests. Along the way they encountered challenges and difficulties. Also discovered support systems and opportunities.

Hadley felt an attraction to the field of nursing. She had always harbored a desire to assist others and make an impact in their lives. Moreover, she possessed a talent for caregiving and healing that was hard to ignore.

Encouraged by her passion she applied to nursing school where she was accepted with arms. She devoted herself wholeheartedly to her studies while skillfully balancing her roles as student, mother and partner. Her determination knew no bounds as she strived to provide her family with a life while realizing her potential.

Upon graduating from nursing school Hadley secured employment at a hospital where she found fulfillment in her work while simultaneously gaining experience.

She developed a passion, for hospice and palliative care dedicating herself to bringing comfort and preserving the dignity of patients during their stages of life. The stories, lessons and wisdom shared by her patients. Motivated her. She formed a connection with them and their families, which led her to pursue a career in this field as her specialization.

Applying to a hospice agency she successfully secured a position. Her role involved providing in home care for patients in their days, weeks or months. Regular visits allowed her to attend to their emotional and spiritual needs while offering support and counseling for their families and loved ones. Witnessing both heart wrenching moments as uplifting encounters left an indelible mark on her. In turn she learned lessons from her patients experiences while imparting knowledge of her own. Participating in their journey was an honor that humbled her.

Chapter 4

Lessons and Legacy

Vlahos is an individual who wears hats. A hospice nurse, an author and a social media influencer. Many know her as "Nurse Hadley" on TikTok, where she shares captivating stories and invaluable insights, from her patients... Her impact goes beyond the realm.

Hadley is also the visionary behind Hadley House, an initiative dedicated to creating an caring environment for families and patients during their final days in hospice care. Her memoir, "The In Between; Unforgettable Encounters During Life's Final Moments " has resonated with readers as it explores how end of life experiences can profoundly shape our perspectives on living.

Drawing from both professional encounters Hadley offers wisdom on life's most profound subjects. Mortality, existence and everything in between. She has immersed herself in research while closely observing the evolving landscape of hospice care not in the United States but also worldwide.

What truly sets Hadley apart is her ability to listen attentively to her patients' stories. Tales of joy, sorrow, love, regret, hopefulness. Which have collectively shaped her understanding of life's intricacies. Through her journey marked by challenges like unplanned pregnancy or divorce alongside moments of love and companionship. She has emerged as an empathetic guide, for others navigating through life's ups and downs. She has also gained insights and wisdom, from her experiences and passions which have shaped her perspective on the complexities of life and death as well as their meaning and purpose.

Hadley offers some reflections and guidance on aspects of life, death and everything in between; Life is a cherished gift that should be embraced wholeheartedly with gratitude. We should never take it for granted. Waste it on matters. Every moment deserves our appreciation. We must seize every opportunity that comes our way. It's vital to stay true to ourselves pursue our dreams and aspirations express love towards those who matter to us and strive to make an impact, on the world.

Death is a part of the cycle of life that shouldn't be feared or avoided. Instead, we should acknowledge its inevitability. Face it with acceptance. Preparing for it by discussing our end-of-life preferences can bring peace of mind. It's equally important to respect others wishes regarding their journey while offering support along the way. Coping with grief allows us to heal while cherishing the memories and legacies left behind by those who have passed away.

The journey between life and death encompasses learning and personal growth. It is crucial not to become stagnant or complacent but instead strive for improvement in ourselves and our lives. Additionally, we should embrace the opportunity to learn from others sharing our stories and wisdom with them. Moreover, we must derive lessons from our experiences overcoming challenges and hardships along the way. Lastly it is important to acknowledge our mistakes learn from them and practice forgiveness towards ourselves and others.

Hadley's profound perspectives on life, death and everything in between hold value not for herself but also for others around her and society as a whole. By utilizing her gift of storytelling, she has managed to touch the hearts of millions of followers and readers with her insights and advice. Furthermore, she has utilized her storytelling abilities to make an impact on the world by supporting movements and causes that deeply resonate with her. Her actions have demonstrated that hospice care is more than a profession; it is a calling that requires both knowledge application as well, as heartfelt dedication.

Hadley Vlahos is a nurse, an author and a social media influencer renowned as "Nurse Hadley" on TikTok. Through her platform she shares heartwarming stories and valuable insights, from her patients. Additionally, Hadley is the visionary behind Hadley House, an initiative that aims to create a nurturing environment for families and patients in their days. She has poured her experiences into the bestselling memoir titled "The In Between; Unforgettable Encounters During Lifes Final Moments' ' which beautifully explores how end of life care can teach us lessons about living.

Hadley's impact on her followers, readers and patients is truly remarkable. Her ability to connect with people both online and in person has left a mark on lives. Through her captivating storytelling she has shared the wisdom. Poignant tales of her patients with millions of followers who have been deeply moved and inspired by her work. Moreover, she has harnessed the power of storytelling to bring about change in society. Lend support to causes close, to her heart. Hadley exemplifies that hospice care encompasses not expertise but also an unwavering vocation driven by compassion and empathy.

Some of the ways Hadley has made an impact and influenced her followers, readers and patients include;

Followers; Hadley has amassed a 1.5 million followers. On this platform she shares videos where she discusses hospice care and shares the lessons and messages, she has received from her patients. Her videos have become sensations attracting millions of views likes, comments and shares. Her followers come from age groups and backgrounds. Many have expressed gratitude, for her work and for sharing her insights. Some have even opened up about their experiences with death and dying seeking advice and support from Hadley.

Through her presence Hadley has fostered a community of individuals interested in hospice care who're willing to have open conversations about death and make plans, for future care. Moreover, she has significantly raised awareness for the importance of hospice care while educating others about its benefits.

Readers; In 2023 Ballantine/Penguin Random House published Hadley's memoir titled "The In Between; Unforgettable Encounters During Life's Final Moments." It became a success by climbing the New York Times bestseller list. The memoir drew inspiration from her TikTok videos. It delved deeper into stories and additional details that she had not previously shared online. It beautifully captured the essence of end-of-life care not imparting lessons about mortality but also shedding light on how to embrace life. Both critics and readers showered the memoir with praise applauding its candor, humor and genuine human touch. The poignant narratives and profound wisdom within the pages sparked conversations and forged connections among readers who found resonance in Hadleys experiences. Through her memoir readers gained insight into the realities faced by those nearing the end of their lives while contemplating the meaning and purpose of life itself.

On her patients; Hadley's role as a hospice nurse has brought her into contact with ill patients and their families. She has provided them with care offering comfort and support to alleviate their pain manage symptoms and navigate through grief. Throughout these encounters she has listened attentively to their stories. Gleaned wisdom from their experiences. Guided by respect, for their wishes and preferences Hadley has guided them on their journey while bringing solace, closure and even moments of joy. Hadley Vlahos has gone above. Beyond, in sharing the stories and wisdom of her patients with an audience. She has truly made an impact on their lives treating them with dignity, respect and providing them with peace.

The influence that Hadley Vlahos has had on her followers, readers and patients is undeniable and commendable. Through her gift of storytelling, she has touched the hearts of millions of people who have been inspired by her work. Moreover, she has utilized her storytelling talent to create a change in society while supporting various social movements and causes close to her heart. Her dedication to hospice care goes beyond being a profession; it is a calling that demands not expertise but also compassion.

Hadley possesses noble aspirations for the future. She aims to further her dedication to hospice care expand her work in this field and make an impact on society. Within the years she has set several goals and formulated plans she is actively pursuing.

Some of her hopes include;

Completing and launching Hadley House, a profit hospice house project that is currently undergoing construction and fundraising efforts. With a focus on promoting comfort and support Hadley envisions an environment where families can be together with their loved ones during their days. Her ultimate goal is to establish a family centered hospice house that fosters gatherings allowing patients to celebrate their lives alongside those to them.

Publishing her book, which will serve as a sequel, to her memoir. This forthcoming publication will center around her experiences in establishing and managing Hadley House.

She desires to share the trials and triumphs of her project involving a hospice house along, with the lessons and messages she received from the families and patients who stayed there. Her aspiration is to inspire and educate others about the significance and advantages of respite care while also encouraging conversations about death and advance care planning.

One of her passions and hobbies is exploring parts of the world. She envisions traveling to destinations across countries immersing herself in cultures and traditions. Additionally, she hopes to visit locations that hold a connection to her work and passion such as hospice houses, death cafes or cemeteries. She has aspirations of learning and evolving through her travels with the intention of sharing her experiences and wisdom with others.

In order to prioritize her family life, which holds a place in her heart she desires to strike a balance between her professional commitments and personal relationships. She aims to savor each moment spent with her family.

Hadley Vlahos' aspirations for the future reflect her dedication and visionary outlook. She yearns to continue expanding upon her work in hospice care making an impact on the world. Simultaneously she seeks fulfillment in nurturing her life and cherishing every moment authentically. Her commitment to hospice care extends beyond being a profession; it is a calling that demands both skillful expertise as well, as heartfelt devotion.

Hadley's expressions of gratitude and appreciation are evident, in aspects of her life and career;

When it comes to her patients and their families Hadley holds gratitude for the trust, they place in her for their care and comfort. She values the opportunity to share in their life experiences, regrets, hopes and wisdom. Hadley commends them for their courage and compassion while respecting their wishes. Supporting them throughout their journey is a privilege she cherishes. Additionally, she shares their stories and wisdom with an audience as a way of honoring their lives impact. She considers these individuals not as patients but as cherished teachers who have imparted lessons about life, death and personal transformation.

Regarding her colleagues and partners; Hadley expresses gratitude for the individuals she has collaborated with on hospice projects and initiatives. She values their shared vision and mission for hospice care. She commends them for their expertise, knowledge, dedication and commitment. Hadley actively collaborates with them to address the challenges that arise in hospice care. She seeks their guidance and input in navigating these obstacles. Furthermore, she forms partnerships with them for events like hospice conferences or publications, through organizations involved in this field. Hadley considers these colleagues as allies who have not contributed to but also enriched her work while providing support and encouragement throughout her journey.

Hadley holds gratitude and appreciation, for her family and friends. She values their love and acceptance well as the support and encouragement they provide in all aspects of her life. She cherishes the time spent together creating memories and expressing love and gratitude towards them. Additionally, Hadley is always there to assist and care for their needs while seeking their support when she requires it. Together they celebrate achievements overcome grief and serve as the pillars that have shaped her character and brought happiness into her life.

Furthermore, Hadley's expression of gratitude extends beyond her circle. She acknowledges the blessings she has received in both interactions with patient's families' followers/readers online colleagues/partners in her profession. Her words and actions reflect an appreciation, for the gifts that life has bestowed upon her. She also shows her thanks and gratitude by dedicating herself to her work and showing compassion. This includes offering comfort, care and support, to her patients and their families. She also shares their stories and wisdom with an audience aiming to make a difference in the world. According to her gratitude and appreciation are aspects of living a life even in the face of death. They are also factors, in finding happiness and fulfillment.

Conclusion

Hadley Vlahos is an individual who has dedicated her life and career to the field of hospice and palliative care. As a registered nurse, author and influential figure, on media she shares her insights and experiences with millions of people. In addition to her pursuits Hadley is a loving wife and mother who gracefully balances the demands of work and family life. She is also the visionary behind Hadley House, a project committed to providing end of life care that upholds dignity for patients and their families.

Hadley's work and message are truly inspiring. Have an impact. She encourages us to cherish and celebrate the moments we share with our loved ones while facing death with courage and serenity. Furthermore, she challenges assumptions around death and dying urging us to embrace the journey in between as a meaningful phase of life. Hadley emphasizes that hospice care encompasses not support but also emotional solace and spiritual guidance.

The biography of Hadley serves as a testament, to her passion, purpose well as the profound significance of hospice care. It is a captivating narrative that resonates deeply within our hearts and minds while prompting introspection about our lives and values.

We must. Rally behind Hadley and her patients offering our support and embracing the opportunity to learn from them as they navigate the challenges of living and facing the end of life gracefully.

www.ingramcontent.com/pod-product-compliance
Lightning Source LLC
Chambersburg PA
CBHW062301290526
45794CB00006B/2644